Essential oils

A quick beginner guide

By Rick Paul

Table of Contents

Introduction

Introduction

I want to thank you and congratulate you for downloading the book, Essential oils.

This book contains proven steps and strategies on how to use Essential oils.

For hundreds of years, essential oils have been used to for various medicinal purposes and lucky for you, they are still here to make your life healthy and awesome. Essential oils are known to combat stress, improve the quality of sleep, fight flu and cold, increase concentration, rid the body of toxins, aid in reducing muscle spasms and reduce chronic pains. Additionally, they are used for cleaning purposes. For instance, Lavender is normally recommended for to relieving stress, banish insomnia and improve the general concentration.

When cooling the skin during hot days is necessary, peppermint essential oil will be handy. Below is an introduction to essential oils on how to use them and why they are the best choice.

Essential oils are hydroponic liquids that are extracted from particular plants and when diluted into the right concentration have healing properties. In recent years essential oils have made their way back into society after having been overlooked for years, mainly due to the modern chemical medicine.

I hope that I have succeeded in making a book that not only is incredibly informative, but also accessible for those who might not have a lot of experience using essential oils.

If you are new to essential oils, you have found the right place. With just a little effort, you will open up an entirely new world of natural solutions to you.

Let's get started!

Chapter 1   What is Essential oils

Essential oils usually are extracted from flowers and also plants, they've been used for many centuries nevertheless remain as valuable things for aromatherapy and also traditional medicinal systems.

There are many of vital oils accessible nowadays, the commonest ones are usually are numbered from 90. An increasing number of are produced so that you can treat illnesses like melanoma, HIV signs and symptoms, asthma, heart strokes along with bronchitis. Essential oils tend to be used with regard to relaxation and massage purposes, but the uses aren't limited.

There are a variety of particular person benefits with regards to the essential oil that is certainly being used as well as the effect from the essential oil depends on where it got their start in.

Why Essential Oils?

It truly is cheaper to work with essential natural oils for household cleaning as compared to using professional cleaning solutions. The essential oils may also be anti-viral, antibacterial, anti-microbial and anti-fungal. They are exceptionally uncomplicated and 100% safe for work with by people coming from all ages and professions.

Essential oils are certainly not only enjoyable and simple to operate, but additionally they work; many people never fail. A few days of employing this products and you're sure of reaping this benefits. Unlike numerous products available on the market that are full of toxins, essential natural oils are non-toxic hence there're safe for the body, the children and actually the pets are certainly not harmed. Of likewise great significance about the use of essential natural oils is they are eco-friendly; at any given time when ecological deterioration worries are therefore high, this is the ideal solution. The extent through which essential oils help the human physical and mental well being is merely remarkable; there're the best substitute for our tribulations.

How to use essential oils.

Just before we commence the talk, it ought to be noted which essential oils usually are not allowed to be directly put on one's skin. In order to become safe, it is strongly recommended that the main oils are generally first diluted. The first task, though, is to test that your skin are not harshly troubled by the fat by assessment it first. This is normally done by simply placing the drop in the oil mixture over a small swatch of the skin. You should leave this particular drop of fat on your skin for at the least 24 hours in order to make certain that you don't have any harmful kind of reaction.

Make sure you include vital oils as part of your daily baths ritual; 8-10 drops added in the bathing water is sufficient to rid the entire body of just about any stress. Lavender, frankincense, roman chamomile, grapefruit in addition to jasmine ought to be in your collection regarding bath moment essential natural skin oils. After a great work out and about, eucalyptus vital oils will likely be great intended for relaxing the muscles in addition to reducing joint pains.

Inhaling vital oils will take your latest mood and provides it a great unimaginable lift up. Experience the magic regarding essential oils in your mood by simply putting 5 in order to 10 drops of the favorite fat in sizzling water. Inhale the steam severally having a towel protected over your brain. Another way to get this done is to put at least 5 drops in the essential oil as part of your dehumidifier; fill your home with fantastic fragrance in addition to relax. For any great goodnight rest, a few drops while on an essential oil around the pillow will work.

How are essential oils extracted?

Essential oils may be extracted while using the distillation method. One process could possibly be steam distillation, the vapor will move upwards over the plant materials causing small oil sacs to be able to rapture and also release their own vapor. Following the oil continues to be extracted, the steam will be combined and cooled and would be condensed. It's going to be separated after which filtered. In addition, there are other processes to have essential natural skin oils like hydro- distillation where inside plant material will likely be boiled in water; this process could be used for flowers.

Why are essential oils effective?

Essential oils carry the ability to protect humans against disease-causing microbes. Many essential oils have been proven to be stimulants or sedatives for humans. The plants were able to adapt to the growing needs of insects and humans, and the essential oil constituents is a proof of this evolution in plants. Human bodies have been biologically programmed to respond to the components of the oils through the receptor sites of the body, the neurochemicals as well as the enzymes that contribute to the benefits of the essential oils.

What essential oils are considered therapeutic?

Tea tree is one good example of an essential oil that can be used to cure a number of illnesses. It can be used for muscle aches and pains and can relieve people from migraine. Other therapeutic oils that can be used for healing will include citrus oils and olive oil.

Chapter 2 Introducing Aromatherapies

Aromatherapy is a kind of alternative medicine, mainly based on essential oils and additional aromatic plant compounds to enhance health as well as mood of the individual. It is also popularly known as Essential Oil Therapy.

Why do People Go after Aromatherapy?

Aromatherapy is totally chemical free and supplement based remedy. Using essential oils within aromatherapy keeps your environment,air pollution free mainly because those essential oils would be the extracts connected with pure herbal products collected in the nature.

For countless years people have put their rely upon several types of essential oils for their therapeutic gains.There will vary ways connected with applying essential oils for aromatherapy with respect to the goals you may need to achieve.

Massage is often a commonly used way of the distribution of aromatherapy gains using essential oils. The rubbing down if done properly by way of a professional counselor can best target the right muscles for optimal gains. But any other person can certainly still find out the art and achieve accomplishment in relaxing tensions along with relieving nervousness. Whether essential oils penetrate the skin or to never achieve any health improvements remains extremely debatable. For many years Aromatherapists claimed that may be how the particular oils treated, but modern-day scientific testing points to the truth that the benefits have been realized by way of inhalation.

Essential Oils for Your Family

Essential oils would be the intense essence of place material, mostly employed in aromatherapy. They may be entirely prepared from botanical matter. They may be mostly confused with all the synthetic perfume oils, which might be chemical regeneration associated with scents prepared mainly via coal tar. Even when the scent of perfume oils could possibly be identical to essential skin oils, they don't get similar element structure and as a consequence, they won't get a similar treatment effect.In fact,the using synthetic perfume oils is restricted to perfumery. Children aromatherapy is a kind of aromatherapy intended to assist throughout, improving the particular happiness and also wellness associated with children.

How to introduce aromatherapy to children

Place 2-3 drops of essential oil on a piece of tissue and keep it close when feeding her or him. This will make the child associate the aroma with comfort and love. You can use this scent during the night to assist the child sleep. When a child is left in a sitter in the presence of aroma, it reassures and comfort her or him.

Use of essential oils in cleaning of children

Children ones like bathtub water, which has a good scent. Roman chamomile and lavender are good selections for youngsters. Use 2-3 drops divorce lawyers Atlanta bath. Citrus oil can be employed as a cleaning agent in the home. Just include few declines of fruit, orange, mandarin or even bergamot fat to drinking water, moisten a sheet of cloth with all the mixture and wipe the children's rooms. Scent the children's drawers keeping the night moment clothing with oil solution put on cotton golf balls. It will deliver the youngsters a sweet dream.

Dosage of essential oil for children

Children respond very well to low dosage of essential oil particularly for irritability and anger. Use a third of adult dosage because their skin is delicate. When adding essential oils to bath water, shake well before blending the correct number of drops with water. Only use those oils safe for children.

Different kinds of Aromatherapy Oils that one should keep at hand

Lavender: It offers a wonderful outside pleasing experiencing. It is often a floral cologne with touch of sweet taste. With calming effect this works question to relax the violent mind. Medicinally, it relieves pain and also minor wounds along with insect hits.

Peppermint: Due to it's one of the main constituents "menthol" it has icy sensation that arouse mental sharpness of the users. Not only that, it sooths migraine, headache, painful muscles, and above all problem of digestion.

Eucalyptus: It is a clean and fresh aroma to open up your congested airways. It is an antibacterial, antimicrobial, antifungal as well as antiinflammatory. It works wonder for asthma, cough and cold, and congestion.

Lemon: It helps to remove bad aura and boost mental alertness. As an antifungal it is wonderful for fixing cuts, cuts, and several other minor injuries. For clearing the air passage, rubbing it on throat and chest will give instant relief.

Tea Tree:. It's famous instead medicine. The astringent on the oil relieves oily secretions over the surface of the skin. The terpinen on the oil soothes little injuries. Contain a little cost you shampoo intended for super cleaning of your respective scalp. Using crucial oils inside aromatherapy may be the latest addition towards cosmetic therapy.

Chapter 3 How does Aromatherapy work

Different ways of uses and applications

Different ways of using essential oils for aromatherapy are widely accepted and many of them optimize inhalation. Depending on the method of application and intended goals, the essential oils are added in just a few drops not exceeding 10% of an ounce (600 drops) of the carrier oil to which they are added. The following are the main categories of uses of different essential oils for different therapeutic method and how they work.

For Skincare

A blend of facial oil can be created by adding up to 15 drops of an essential oil to a carrier oil of choice, unscented lotion or cream. Rosemary is one of the essential oils that can be added to a skin cream to help in rewinding the aging clock. Facial steam for skincare and cleansing routines requires about 5 drops added in a facial steam or a pint of water that is warm. 5 drops of a favorite essential oil can be added to honey, egg white, moistened clay or mashed avocado, for facial masks. For the entire body use, add 3 drops of an essential oil like pink grapefruit that can simulate to the bristles of a bath brush. You can brush from your toes or fingers towards the heart to experience the stimulating effect.

For treatment

Inhalation is probably the best ways involving using essential natural oils for treatment involving problems like sinus or bronchial illnesses. You can add about drops for you to steaming water in a bowl. You are able to capture the steam by using a towel for inhaling while your sight remain closed before the oil smell diminishes. The procedure is usually repeated every 5 hrs if necessary. Up to 9 fat drops can also be added to a humidifier's water after which left running immediately. A nebulizer via microdiffusion produces micro-particles of your essential in their particular millions to optimize the effect of inhalation regarding treatment. Adding gas drops to normal water in bath tubs, Jacuzzi, showers and for easy use in topical applications is additionally meant for treatment of numerous ailments.

For household uses

When cleaning different surfaces around the house, essential oils can be used with various detergents and soaps. They will leave behind their fragrances and continue to provide the benefits of aromatherapy for hours. They can be used when doing laundry, washing dishes, flavoring and general cleaning.

How Essential Oils Work to Relieve the Patients?

Aromatic or Essential oils stimulate the olfactory nerves from the patients along with send signals for the Neuro-receptors in your brain. It is a result of this reason that after you employ them a good electro-chemical answer is induced that promotes the total amount in your nervous process and aid relieving hassles. Though there are many of man-made aromatic oils you can buy that amount to less. Yet, these oils aren't recommended. For top results, use certified crucial oils which can be free by pesticides.

Do fragrant healing soy candles truly work?

All over again, fragrant healing may be utilized by individuals everywhere internationally since the starting of development. It might become tricky to contend against the viability of the practice regardless to the fact that its belongings have been totally psychosomatic. Inside correlation, western medication offers just barely did start to understand the adequacy or maybe fragrance based treatment.

Fragrance based treatment utilizes the inbuilt mending forces of the pith or stench of specific plant life, blooms, roots, etc. A standard lighting scented with counterfeit aroma won't have the same effect. The explanation behind it is on the reasons that fundamental herbal oils are inferred from common sources although consistently scented luminous made of wax utilizes chemicals in order to copy certain fragrances. The body is aware of which aroma can be common and that fragrance is constructed.

When you light a typical scented candle, you merely about quickly start to smell the perfume being discharged because of the scent or aroma that may be imbued with the flame wax. In the event you are useful to the solid, impactful aromas connected with current scented candle lights, it may take that you while to stench the fragrance being discharged with a fragrant healing soy luminous made of wax.

The contrasts involving a fragrance misleadingly processed by an aroma along with a smell regularly earned by and critical oil are considerable. Scent fragrances are generally helpful in that they can trigger memory receptors as well as subsequently influence tendency. Nonetheless, crucial oils handle this level and a noticeably much deeper degree. It is not so much the aroma from the key oil that may be helpful. It happens to be accepted that the chemicals in these oils possess a measurable impact within the physical body.

It's always best to utilize soy wax when making use of key plant oils for a few reasons. Firstly, it blazes neatly and doesn't antagonistically influence the scent of the crucial oils. It likewise blazes cooler, which permits the scent being scattered even more gradually and even more equally, in supplement, the oils aren't warmed up to the point where the critical oils are damaged. This can take place with paraffin given it smolders sultrier as well as producing carbon based sediment when blazed.

On the point when using a fragrant healing soy luminous made of wax, it is prescribed that you simply discover a relaxed spot to sit and breathe in the fragrance for no less than a half hr. This will supply the vital oils time to communicate using your body.

The general uses of Aromatherapy

Aromatherapy is used generally for flu, colds, sore muscles, relaxation etc.

Bath: If you use this therapy for bathing, then fill the tub and add essential oils. In addition, to take a small cup of milk and add the oils with a tablespoon of honey and then add it into the water.

Shower: After a shower, take five to seven drops of essential oils on a damp, clean cloth and then rub it on the whole body. After that, allow it to dry in the air.

Compress: This therapy is excellent for lessening the pain. This oil is useful for menstrual cramps or strained muscles, etc. Add four to seven drops of Essential Oil into a bowl of water. Take a cloth, dip it into the water and wring it out. Now place the cloth on the painful area. Repeat it, when the cloth cools. A plastic sheet or towel can be covered on the warm cloth. It will help to keep the warm for long time. This therapy is very much helpful for getting relief from menstrual cramps.

Jacuzzi: If you go after bath tub or Jacuzzi, then add 3 drops of essential oil for an individual. You can repeat it after every 30 minutes. But remember that a few essential oil can damage the plastic tub.

Bath salts: Take some Epsom salts, baking soda and sea salt and mix them well. Then add six to ten drops essential oil with this mixture and blend it well. You can add it with warm water for bathe or can rub this blend before the bath.It helps to cure aching muscle or sore.

Chapter 4 List of common oils and their uses

Here are some of the essential oils used for weight loss:

Grapefruit Oil:

Grapefruit oil naturally suppresses the appetite through a process known as lipolysis. It also dissolves fats. It combines very well with lavender in a Whiffer aromatherapy pendant.

Peppermint Oil:

Peppermint oil helps one to feel fuller. It actually affects the part of the brain that deals with satiety or feeling full. Dr. Alan Hirsch of the Smell and Taste Treatment and Research Institute of Chicago recommends that inhaling the aroma of these essential oils throughout the day and before each meal can greatly help to curb appetite.

Tangerine Oil:

Tangerine essential oil is another citrus-based oil that may help with weight loss. It also helps to regulate metabolism, create a feeling of happiness and reduce anxiety. However, one should not go out in the sun after applying tangerine oil. It is often combined with bergamot or lavender.

Vanilla Oil:

Vanilla essential oils might help curb the desire for food for sweets which can be very common throughout women. They can be used in a diffuser or maybe in aromatherapy candles to aid curb cravings. Reducing the volume of sweets in one's diet regime can go a considerable ways towards significant weight loss and reducing the danger of diabetes.

Bergamot Oil:

Bergamot oil doesn't directly curb hunger but has soothing effects within the mind. It basically eliminates stress and creates an awareness of of well-being. Dr. Hirsch recommends that bergamot could be combined with lavender oil which has calming properties. Owing to the truth that people tend to consume more when there're stressed, smelling bergamot oil can establish a sense connected with calmness that continues them from eating once they are not truly hungry.

Patchouli Oil:

Patchouli essential oil can help to effectively control appetite. It can also be used as a sedative and relaxation aid. These oils can be used in a bath or in a diffuser. When used in a bath, 10 -15 drops of the oil should be added to the bath water. Patchouli works more effectively in the evening hours. When used in a diffuser, the same amount should be added to an oil diffuser and inhaled deeply.

Rose Geranium Oil:

Rose geranium is a very powerful essential oil with mood lifting qualities. It therefore reduces appetite which results in one eating less food.

Ylang ylang Oil:

Used to clarify thoughts and assist in a feeling of wellness and calm. It therefore curbs appetite resulting to consumption of less food.

Dill Oil

This oil is extracted from dill seeds and has sedative properties. It does not contain cholesterol and low in calories. It therefore effectively contributes to weight loss.

Orange Oil:

Helps overcome depression and gives emotional support.

Essential oils will help in weight-loss through which affects one's disposition. Depression and stress tend to be the reasons behind overeating. Using the calming vital oils such as lavender regarding massage and bath will help relax the entire body, improve your mood therefore eliminate some of the psychological causes for overeating.

Here are the essential oils used for a quick relieve from headaches:

Lavender Oil:

Lavender oil is probably the most well-liked and low-priced essential herbal oils for head ache relieve out there. It incorporates a high percent of esters and hence it provides antiinflammatory and also sedative components. It encourages relation, helps someone to sleep and also treats headaches and depression symptoms. Lavender oil works better when employed to alleviate headaches at night time hours.

Jasmine Oil:

Though it's a bit more expensive than other essential oils, Jasmine oil has therapeutic properties that are very strong hence making it very valuable. This oil provides energy and calms emotions at the same time. It also improves the tone of a person's skin. A wide range of Sandalwood, Bergamot, Rose and citrus oils can be blended with Jasmine very effectively.

Chamomile Oil:

Both Roman and German Chamomile oil have powerful properties that can be used to treat premenstrual syndrome which is a major cause of headache. Chamomile has also been recommended by health practitioners to calm severe headache resulting from irritability. It can be blended in massage oil or a few drops can be placed in a bath, vaporizer or diffuser.When combined with creams and lotions, Chamomile becomes more efficient for headache relieve.

Rose Oil:

Just like Jasmine, Rose is a multipurpose fat. It's normally blended with other crucial oils such as Bergamot, patchouli, cedarwood, chamomile and also sandalwood. It can be utilized for anti-depressant to generate feelings associated with calmness. Since trauma is a common reason for severe headaches, this oil can promote over emotional healing on this condition. Rose oil for headaches may be added in order to massage fat or bath tub product.

Eucalyptus oil:

Eucalyptus radiata and Eucalyptus globules contain a significant amount of oxide 1, 8-Cineole. 1, 8-Cineole acts as both an expectorant as well as an antiinflammatory. Eucalyptus oil helps to ease headaches especially those associated with sinus headaches.

Taking Care of Your Skin with Essential Oils

Tea Tree Oil

Tea tree oil is usually an alternate prestigious oil around the grounds it has outstanding medicinal components, for illustration, antibacterial, antiviral, antifungal, germicide and also pain reduce. Thusly they have the beautiful abilities to extract, clean, and also sooth chafed, aroused skin conditions. It is actually quick acting and may clear way up skin inflammation, flaws and also pimples rapidly.

Sandalwood oil

Sandalwood should be to a fantastic degree saturating oil that is certainly useful to get dried out or dried out skin. Sandalwood may evacuate lines and wrinkles, scars, in addition to almost minimal differences. It truly is likewise a antibacterial in addition to antifungal which often can lessen the wedding of pimple inflammation in addition to skin ailments.

Lemon oil

Lemon oil and different citrus oils are extraordinary for clearing up pimple inflammation quick by evacuating the abundance sebum and oil on the face. It has extraordinary recuperating and remedial qualities particularly when connected to healthy skin. Lemon oil can light up ones composition by evacuating dead skin cells. Be that as it may, it can result in skin staining when laid open to steer daylight, accordingly it's basic to stay out of the sun instantly in the wake of applying lemon oil.

Clary Sage Oil

Clary sage is advantageous for skin conditions are produced by hormone lopsided attributes, for illustration, pimple infection, wrinkles along with barely incomparable differences. Clary Sage has a comparative structure to human being hormones coupled these lines maybe it's utilized to be able to supplement with regard to imbalanced bodily hormones when uncovered into the body. It furthermore goes about being an antibacterial along with astringent to be able to murder contamination along with purge acute wounds.

Myrrh Oil

Myrrh oil has been utilized for a long time and within aged times utilized as a part of an emollient to treat just about any illness. It has been known to treat dry skin, wrinkles, rashes, imperfections, dermatitis, and microscopic organisms in the skin.

Natural Essential Oil Based Hair Care Products

List of Essential Oils

Lavender Oil: it has proven hair benefits and works well for all hair types. Lavender oil is a good treatment for itching and dandruff and it is helpful in improving hair growth and controlling hair breakage.

Chamomile Oil: is known to soothe the hair and scalp, and helps to retract inflamed skin cells, to alleviate dandruff conditions and itching scaly scalp.

Peppermint Oil: helps to nourish the hair by stimulating blood flow to the hair root.

Rosemary Oil: is useful for flaky itchy scalp and dandruff problems.

Tea Tree Oil: it helps to keep the scalp free of fungal problems and bacteria and it is a great moisturizer for the hair.

Lemon Oil: is beneficial for oily hair and it is recommended for dandruff and lice.

Myrrh Oil: is very good for dry hair and dandruff.

Carrier Oils

Carrier oils are another type of oils for hair that can help carry the essential oil onto the skin. They are derived from nuts or seeds by maceration or cold pressing. Carrier oils are nourishing the hair and they are great moisturizers and strengtheners.

Oils for Normal Hair

These essential oils are working best for normal hair:

- Clary Sage

- Rosemary

- Cedar wood

- Thyme

- Lemon

- Lavender

- Geranium

The best carrier oils to use for normal hair are almond, jojoba, and borage.

Chapter 5   Recipe

Recipe for Skin Moisturizing Lotion

This recipe is essentially for a great skin moisturizing lotion for everybody:

Ingredients

- 15 drops of natural Geranium
- 8 lotion base ounces
- 5 drops of ylang ylang
- 10 drops of some myrrh

Procedure

Before you start to make your skin layer care blend, it is significant to note that you ought to always use therapeutically pure grade essential oils. The procedure is simply adding essential oils into a lotion in addition to mixing the mixture lightly. Add the label that contains the substances you utilised in the box.

Myrrh in addition to geranium usually are some typical essential oils which have been used extensively to heal your skin. Adding ylang ylang will simply improve the oils fragrance, which is often a very recipe will cool in addition to soften skin and have tried them in cleaning some unsightly stains from hands and wrists. key theory to aromatherapy regarding consumers. If customers do not like the aroma they will also steer clear of buying the goods. This is simply an illustration of this what you can use, there vary combinations offered.

For skins which have been so dried up, it is significant to increase 10 declines of Roman Chamomile, Rose and Sandalwood in order to one's 8 oz of bottom lotion. Be sure only pure therapeutic essential grade natural oils are largely used.

If an example may be so much thinking about making their very own lotion make use of by introducing some essential oils, then this old recipe will cool in addition to soften skin and have tried them in cleaning some unsightly stains from hands and wrists.

Ingredients

- 1 ounce freshly squeezed lemon juice
- 1 ounce of rosewater
- 10 therapeutic grade essential oils of choice
- 1 ounce of glycerin

Procedure

Put all this items in a clean bottle and shake them gently. Label the bottle with some instructions of shaking well before any use and label all the ingredients used on the outside of the bottle, and then store them in a clean refrigerator. This mixture needs to be used for a maximum of three weeks, hence, require one to use them in small amounts at one particular time.

Recipe for a Winter Lotion

Ingredients

- Half a cup of rose water or distilled water

- 1 tablespoonful of lecithin

- Half a cup of jojoba oil

- 1 vitamin E capsule

- 15 drops of one's favorite essential oils therapeutic grade

Procedure

Put all the products not including vitamins At the capsule inside a blender as well as whip these people until these people form a fine nice cream. Feel liberated to add more distilled water when you really need a slimmer lotion. Add oil and e vitamin capsule at the end of it. Lecithin is often a mixing agent that aids water as well as oil adhere together. Mix them all well as store these people in quite clean storage units labeled along with ingredients utilized.

Cream oil is often a particular vegetable oil that's some water put into it. This particular however, is an ideal skin color moisturizer.Cream is thicker as compared to lotion oil mainly because it has much less water. The persistence of almost any lotion helps make the lotion suited to oily or perhaps normal skin color. Cream has the spreading easiness for the skin and does not leave greasy coats onto it. Adding vital oils for you to skin will certainly enhance making use of essential natural skin oils for skin care therapeutic benefit.

Conclusion

Thank you again for downloading this book!

I hope this book was able to help you to know about   Essential   oils.

Finally, if you enjoyed this book, then I'd like to ask you for a favor, would you be kind enough to leave a review for this book on Amazon? It'd be greatly appreciated!

Thank you and good luck!

www.ingramcontent.com/pod-product-compliance
Lightning Source LLC
Chambersburg PA
CBHW071153280526
45787CB00003B/1500